PREVENTION AND MANAGEMENT OF CHRONIC LOWER RESPIRATORY DISEASE

The Comprehensive Guide To
Prevent And Manage Chronic
Lower Respiratory Diseases
By
Patricia J. Taylor

PREFACE

With an estimated 3.2 million deaths per year, chronic lower respiratory diseases are one of the leading causes of death in the world today. Surprisingly few people are aware of these diseases and how to prevent and manage them, despite the enormous burden they place on people, families, healthcare systems, and societies.

This book aims to fill that knowledge gap by giving readers a thorough understanding of chronic lower respiratory diseases, their causes, and preventative measures. It provides useful guidance on how to spot risk factors, stop disease progression, and control symptoms. It also offers guidance on how to access the support and services needed to improve the quality of life for those living with the conditions.

This book is for anyone seeking to understand chronic lower respiratory diseases and the steps needed to prevent and manage them. It is for those living with the conditions, their families and caregivers, health care professionals, and all individuals interested in improving public health and reducing the burden of these diseases.

We grow to admire the bravery and tenacity of those who battle chronic lower respiratory diseases as we learn more about their complexities. We also start to understand how crucial it is to work together to create better treatments and achieve better results.

We hope that this book serves as an inspiration and a guide for those who are determined to make a difference in the fight against these debilitating diseases. This book is meant to contribute to that effort.

Thank you for taking the time to read this book and for joining us in the effort to prevent and manage chronic lower respiratory diseases.

Sincerely,
Patricia J. Taylor

Table of Contents

PREFACE

Table of Contents

INTRODUCTION
  Definition
  Prevalence
  Types of chronic lower respiratory diseases
  Causes of chronic lower respiratory diseases

RISK FACTORS AND PREVENTION
  Common Risk Factors:
  Strategies To Prevention

DIAGNOSIS AND TREATMENT
  Diagnostic Tests
  Medical Tests

HOMECARE AND LIFESTYLE MODIFCATION
  Nutrition And Exercise

Managing Stress And Fatigue

MANAGEMENT OF CHRONIC LOWER RESPIRATORY
Medications
Oxygen Therapy
Pulmonary Rehabilitation

COPING STRATEGIES FOR CHRONIC LOWER RESPIRATORY DISEASES
Complementary And Alternative Therapy (CAM)

RESOURCES AND SUPPORT
Exercising Tips To Follow For People With CLRD
A 7-Day Meal Plan For People Living With CLRD

CONCLUSION

INTRODUCTION

Do you ever feel like you can't catch your breath? That can be a scary feeling, especially when it happens often. Unfortunately, it's a reality for many people who suffer from chronic lower respiratory diseases. These diseases can cause difficulty breathing, tightness in the chest, and even coughing.

Chronic respiratory diseases are a global health concern, affecting millions of people around the world. These diseases can range from asthma to chronic obstructive pulmonary disease (COPD) and can have a significant impact on day-to-day life. It is estimated that between 5-10% of the world's population suffers from some form of chronic respiratory disease, making it one of the leading causes of death and disability worldwide. It is important to recognize the burden of these diseases and prioritize strategies to reduce their occurrence. This article will provide an overview of chronic respiratory diseases, their causes, and available treatments, as well as discuss strategies to reduce their prevalence and improve the quality of life of those affected.

By understanding the risk factors and symptoms associated with chronic respiratory diseases, we can take steps to reduce the occurrence of these diseases and improve the quality of life of those affected. Through early diagnosis and appropriate treatment, we can provide a better outlook for those affected by these conditions, and support them to lead healthier and more fulfilling lives.

So, let's take a look at what chronic lower respiratory diseases are, how they affect people, and what you can do if you think you or someone you know might be suffering from one of these conditions.

Definition

Chronic lower respiratory diseases (CLRD) is a group of diseases that affect the airways and other structures of the lungs, causing the lungs to be unable to provide the necessary oxygen to the body. These diseases, which include asthma, chronic bronchitis, emphysema, and chronic obstructive pulmonary disease (COPD), can lead to serious health complications and, if left untreated, can be life-threatening.

The most common symptoms of chronic lower respiratory diseases are difficulty breathing, coughing, wheezing, and chest tightness. Treatment for these conditions often includes medications, lifestyle changes, and other therapies to help reduce symptoms and improve quality of life.

Prevalence

Lower chronic respiratory diseases are a common condition that affects millions of people worldwide. According to the World Health Organization, an estimated 235 million people suffer from the chronic obstructive pulmonary disease (COPD) and an estimated 334 million people suffer from asthma. COPD is the fourth leading cause of death globally and is expected to become the third leading cause of death by 2030. In the United States, COPD affects more than 11 million adults and is the third leading cause of death. Asthma affects an estimated 7 million adults and 6 million children in the United States and is the most common chronic condition among children.

The prevalence of lower chronic respiratory diseases is influenced by a variety of factors including age, gender, lifestyle, genetics, environment, and social determinants such as income and education. In addition, smoking is a major risk factor for lower chronic respiratory diseases, particularly COPD. Poor air quality, both indoors and outdoors, is also a major contributor to the prevalence of lower chronic respiratory diseases.

The burden of lower chronic respiratory diseases is significant and is likely to continue to rise as the population ages and environmental conditions worsen. As such, it is important to focus on reducing the risk factors associated with lower chronic respiratory diseases, as well as increasing access to diagnosis and treatment.

Types of chronic lower respiratory diseases

Chronic lower respiratory diseases (CLRD) are a group of diseases that affect the lower airways of the lungs, including the trachea, bronchi, and bronchioles. These diseases can cause symptoms such as coughing, shortness of breath, chest tightness, and difficulty breathing. Below are the types of CLRD:

Chronic obstructive pulmonary disease (COPD) is a progressive lung illness that makes breathing difficult. It is brought on by prolonged exposure to irritants such as dust, fumes from chemicals, and cigarette smoke. Emphysema and chronic bronchitis are the two primary forms of COPD. Shortness of breath, a chronic cough, and weariness are all signs of COPD.

Asthma is a chronic inflammatory disorder of the airways that can cause symptoms such as wheezing, coughing, and chest tightness. It is caused by environmental triggers, such as dust, pollen, and air pollution. Asthma can be managed with medications and lifestyle changes.

There are some illnesses collectively known as interstitial lung disease (ILD) that result in lung inflammation and scarring. It is usually caused by long-term exposure to irritants, such as asbestos and coal dust. Symptoms of ILD include shortness of breath, chest pain, and a dry cough.

Bronchitis is an inflammation of the bronchial tubes that carry air to and from the lungs. It is usually caused by a viral infection, but can also be caused by environmental factors such as air pollution or smoking. Symptoms include coughing, chest pain, and difficulty breathing.

Mycobacterium tuberculosis is the bacterium that causes the lung condition known as tuberculosis. More than 1.8 billion people around the world have tuberculosis, but the disease is only considered active in 10 million of them.

People with strong immune systems sometimes carry an inactive form of the disease, called latent tuberculosis. In people with weaker immune systems, the bacteria attack lung tissue. It can also spread and cause damage to other parts of the body.

An infection of the lungs known as pneumonia is brought on by bacteria, viruses, or fungi. Symptoms include fever, chills, chest pain, and difficulty breathing. It can be treated with antibiotics and antiviral medications.

Cystic fibrosis is an inherited disorder that affects the lungs and other organs. It is characterized by the buildup of thick, sticky mucus in the lungs and other organs, which can lead to difficulty breathing, coughing, and an increased risk of infection. Treatment includes medications, airway clearance techniques, and lung transplantation.

Pulmonary fibrosis is a condition in which the lung tissue becomes thick and stiff, resulting in difficulty breathing. It is usually caused by long-term exposure to environmental toxins, certain medications, or a viral infection. Medication, oxygen therapy, and lifestyle modifications are all part of the treatment.

Lung cancer is one of the most common cancers in the US, with more than 218,000 cases, ranking third overall. It can develop as either small-cell lung cancer or non-small-cell lung cancer, which is the more common of the two.

Emphysema is a type of chronic lower respiratory disease that is characterized by damage to the air sacs (alveoli) in the lungs. This damage causes the walls of the air sacs to weaken and break down, allowing air to get trapped in the lungs. This trapped air makes it difficult for the lungs to fully expand and contract, causing shortness of breath and difficulty breathing. Emphysema is often caused by long-term exposure to air pollutants, such as cigarette smoke, and can lead to an increased risk of other respiratory conditions, such as bronchitis and asthma. Treatment for emphysema typically involves medications and lifestyle changes, such as quitting smoking, to help reduce symptoms and slow the progression of the disease.

These diseases often require long-term management and lifestyle changes to reduce symptoms and improve quality of life.

Causes of chronic lower respiratory diseases

Numerous microbes, such as bacteria, viruses, and fungi, are responsible for lower respiratory infections.

Lower respiratory diseases are typically caused by viral pathogens, which include rhinoviruses, respiratory syncytial viruses, influenza, parainfluenza, human metapneumovirus, measles, mumps, adenoviruses, and coronaviruses.

Bacterial pathogens are less common than viral but can include Streptococcus pneumoniae, Mycoplasma pneumoniae, Haemophilus influenzae, and Chlamydophila pneumoniae. Coxiella burnetii and Legionella pneumophila can cause outbreaks and sporadic cases of respiratory illness. A secondary viral respiratory infection may also result in bacterial sinusitis, bronchitis, or pneumonia.

Other Causes:

Environmental hazards: Certain environmental hazards, such as secondhand smoke and air pollution, can cause chronic lower respiratory diseases.

Autoimmune diseases: Autoimmune diseases, such as rheumatoid arthritis and lupus, can cause chronic lower respiratory diseases.

RISK FACTORS AND PREVENTION

Common Risk Factors:

There are two major risk factors for lower respiratory diseases. As follows:

Genetics can play a role in the development and progression of chronic lower respiratory diseases. Genetic factors can affect an individual's susceptibility to environmental exposures as well as how well they will react to and recover from the exposure. While some genes may protect against environmental toxins, others may make people more susceptible to respiratory illnesses. The way a person will develop a specific respiratory illness or how severe the illness will be can also be influenced by genetic variations. Moreover, certain genetic mutations have been connected to specific respiratory illnesses, including cystic fibrosis and chronic obstructive pulmonary disease (COPD).

The risk of lower respiratory illnesses may run in some families. For instance, those with cystic fibrosis may be more likely to get bronchitis and lung infections.

As a result, those who have a family history of these illnesses may be more likely to contract them. It is significant to remember that, although environmental exposures can play a role in the development of respiratory diseases, genetics can also be a risk factor.

Environmental factors are a major risk factor for chronic lower respiratory diseases (CLRD). These diseases are caused by a combination of genetic and environmental factors.

When environmental factors are considered risk factors for CLRD, there are several important factors to consider.

Smoking is the most common and important risk factor for CLRD. Cigarette smoking is responsible for about 80-90% of deaths from COPD and is a major risk factor for all other CLRD. Even secondhand smoke can increase the risk of developing CLRD, especially in children. Both active and passive exposure to tobacco smoke can cause inflammation and damage to the airways, which can lead to the development or worsening of CLRD.

The second is air pollution. Air pollution is the presence of pollutants in the air, such as particulate matter, ozone, and nitrogen dioxide. These pollutants can irritate the airways and lead to inflammation, which can trigger asthma symptoms or worsen existing CLRD.

Third, the presence of allergens or irritants in the home environment can also trigger asthma symptoms or worsen existing CLRD. Common allergens and irritants include dust mites, mold, pet dander, and cockroach droppings.

Fourth, occupational exposures can also increase the risk of developing or exacerbating CLRD. Occupational exposures include exposure to dust, gases, smoke, and other chemicals.

Finally, the climate and weather can also increase the risk of developing or exacerbating CLRD. High temperatures, humidity, and air pollution levels can all trigger asthma symptoms or worsen existing CLRD.

Environmental factors are a major risk factor for CLRD and should not be overlooked. Reducing exposure to environmental pollutants and allergens, avoiding secondhand smoke, and limiting occupational exposures are all important steps to reduce the risk of developing or exacerbating CLRD.

Other Risk Factors are :

Age is also a risk factor for CLRD. As people get older, the risk of developing CLRD increases.

Gender: Men are more likely to develop chronic lower respiratory diseases than women.

Obesity: People who are overweight or obese are more likely to develop CLRD. Excess weight puts added strain on the lungs, which increases the risk of developing CLRD.

People with other respiratory or cardiovascular conditions are also at greater risk of developing CLRD.
Conditions such as Lung Cancer , Lung infections , Autoimmune diseases, such as rheumatoid arthritis and lupus and heart disease can increase the risk of CLRD.

Weakened Immune System: People with weakened immune systems, such as those who are HIV positive, are at an increased risk of developing lower respiratory diseases. This is because their bodies are unable to fight off infections and diseases, such as pneumonia, as effectively as healthy individuals.

Strategies To Prevention

Smoking Cessation
A multifaceted strategy including quitting smoking, vaccination, better air quality, lifestyle changes, early diagnosis, and treatment of pre-existing conditions is needed to prevent chronic lower respiratory diseases (CLRD).

One of the most crucial elements in the prevention of chronic lower respiratory diseases is smoking cessation, which is the process of quitting smoking. Smoking cessation can help reduce the risk of developing chronic lower respiratory diseases such as COPD (Chronic Obstructive Pulmonary Disease), asthmatic bronchitis, and emphysema.

For those who have a family history of chronic lower respiratory diseases, quitting smoking is especially crucial. According to estimates, quitting smoking can cut a person's risk of COPD by half. Asthma and chronic bronchitis are two other chronic lower respiratory illnesses that can be prevented or treated by quitting smoking.

Numerous methods, including medication, counseling, support groups, and nicotine replacement therapy, are available to people who want to stop smoking. In addition to counseling, medications like bupropion and varenicline can help reduce cravings by reducing nicotine withdrawal symptoms. Nicotine replacement therapy can ease the discomfort brought on by withdrawal symptoms, and support groups can offer social support and encouragement.

To lower the risk of chronic lower respiratory diseases, it's crucial to adopt new lifestyle habits in addition to these prevention methods. Getting regular exercise, eating well, and abstaining from secondhand smoke can all help lower the risk of contracting these illnesses.

Vaccination
Many chronic lower respiratory diseases, including chronic obstructive pulmonary disease (COPD), bronchitis, and asthma, can be prevented with vaccination. Vaccines can offer defense against a variety of infectious agents and are particularly useful in preventing serious, potentially fatal illnesses. Children, adolescents, and adults are typically given vaccinations to protect them from specific infections.

Vaccines work by introducing a weakened or otherwise harmless form of a virus or bacteria into the body. In other words, if the person is exposed to the disease, their body will be better able to fight it off. This helps the body develop an immunity to the disease. Vaccines can also be used to treat certain illnesses or infections more effectively or even to stop them from happening altogether. For example, the measles, mumps, and rubella (MMR) vaccine can help prevent the development of measles, mumps, and rubella.

Additionally, vaccines can aid in preventing some chronic lower respiratory illnesses like COPD, asthma, and bronchitis. For instance, the pneumococcal vaccine can aid in preventing infection from a specific strain of Streptococcus pneumoniae that can result in pneumonia and other serious illnesses. The influenza vaccine can also help to reduce the severity and incidence of certain respiratory illnesses, particularly in older adults who are more at risk of developing serious complications from the flu.

Overall, vaccination is the best defense against chronic lower respiratory diseases for both you and your loved ones. Vaccines are safe, and effective, and can help to prevent serious and potentially life-threatening illnesses. The best vaccines for you and your family should be discussed with your doctor or other healthcare providers.

Improved Air Quality

Improved air quality is a key prevention tool for reducing chronic lower respiratory diseases. Poor air quality can contain pollutants such as particulate matter, ozone, and other pollutants that can exacerbate the symptoms of respiratory diseases. These pollutants can also cause inflammation in the lungs, which can lead to long-term health problems. We can reduce the number of pollutants that enter our lungs and the risk of developing chronic lower respiratory diseases by improving air quality.

To improve air quality, governments and organizations can take several steps. The most important is reducing the number of air pollutants released into the air. This can be accomplished through the use of cleaner-burning fuels, such as natural gas and renewable energy sources. The use of catalytic converters in vehicles can also reduce emissions of pollutants such as carbon monoxide, nitrogen oxides, and hydrocarbons. Additionally, the implementation of stringent emission standards, such as the European Union's Euro 5 and Euro 6 standards, can help reduce emissions from vehicles and industrial sources.

Another way to improve air quality is to reduce the amount of dust and smoke particles in the air. This can be done by regularly cleaning and dusting the home and workplace, using air filters, and avoiding smoking indoors.

Another strategy for improving air quality is through the use of green spaces. Green spaces, such as parks and forests, can reduce the concentration of pollutants in the air by acting as a filter. They also reduce the heat island effect, which can cause a rise in temperatures in urban areas. Additionally, they can reduce levels of noise pollution.

Finally, improved air quality can be achieved through public education and awareness campaigns. These campaigns can educate the public on the dangers of air pollution and how to reduce their exposure to it. For example, people can be encouraged to use other healthcare providersalk or cycle instead of driving, and wear protective masks when air pollution levels are high.

In summary, Improving air quality is an important prevention tool to reduce the risk of chronic lower respiratory diseases. By reducing the number of pollutants entering the atmosphere and reducing dust and smoke particles in the air, we can help ensure better air quality and reduce the risk of respiratory diseases.

Other Strategies For Prevention are

1. Lifestyle Changes: One of the most important strategies for CLRD prevention is to modify lifestyle habits that contribute to the development of the condition. This includes avoiding alcohol consumption, eating a healthy diet, and engaging in regular physical activity. Additionally, individuals should be aware of their risk factors for CLRD and take steps to reduce them, such as controlling blood sugar levels and managing asthma.

2. Early Diagnosis: Early diagnosis of CLRD is crucial to preventing the progression of the disease. This includes being aware of the signs and symptoms of CLRD and seeking medical attention if they occur. Additionally, individuals should also be aware of the risk factors for CLRD and get regular check-ups to detect any early signs of the condition.

3. Treatment of Existing Conditions: Treatment of existing conditions is essential to prevent the progression of CLRD. This includes managing and controlling any underlying conditions that may contribute to the development of CLRD, such as asthma or COPD. Additionally, medications that reduce inflammation of the airways and improve airflow can help prevent the progression of the disease.

DIAGNOSIS AND TREATMENT

Diagnostic Tests

Chronic lower respiratory diseases can have serious long-term effects, so early diagnosis and treatment are key to managing these conditions. Diagnostic tests play an important role in diagnosing and managing these conditions. These tests can help determine the severity of the disease, the presence of any complications, and the best course of treatment. The best way to diagnose chronic lower respiratory diseases is through a combination of diagnostic tests.

The first step in diagnosing CLRD is to take a detailed medical history, including any past diagnosis, symptoms, and exposures to a doctor if you suspect that you have any CLRD.

The doctor may also perform a physical exam. During this exam, the doctor will listen to the patient's lungs and look for signs of inflammation or obstruction in the respiratory system. The doctor may also use a stethoscope to listen for crackles and wheezing, which can be signs of airway obstruction.

In addition to the physical exam, there are several diagnostic tests that can be used to evaluate chronic lower respiratory diseases. These tests include spirometry, chest X-ray, CT scan and bronchoscopy.

Spirometry is a test that measures how much air a person can breathe in and out. It can help diagnose asthma and other obstructive lung diseases such as COPD. The test involves having the patient blow into a tube or machine, which measures the amount of air they can exhale in one second.

The most common form of diagnostic test used to diagnose chronic lower respiratory diseases is a chest X-ray. This type of test can provide detailed images of the lungs, which can help to detect any abnormal shapes or sizes and any evidence of other conditions such as cysts or tumors. Additionally, a chest X-ray can show if there are any changes in the shape or size of the lungs, which can be indicative of a chronic lower respiratory disease.

Another important diagnostic test for chronic lower respiratory diseases is a pulmonary function test. This type of test measures the amount of air that can be exhaled from the lungs and the amount of oxygen that is present in the air that is inhaled. This type of test can help to determine how well the lungs are functioning and can be useful in diagnosing certain chronic lower respiratory diseases.

In addition to these two tests, a doctor may also order a CT scan of the lungs. This type of scan can provide detailed images of the lungs, which can help to detect any abnormalities or blockages in the airways. It can also be used to detect any signs of infection or inflammation that may be present in the lungs, which can be indicative of a chronic lower respiratory disease.

Finally, a bronchoscopy is a procedure in which a small camera is inserted into the airways of the lungs. This type of test can help to detect any abnormalities or blockages in the airways, which can be indicative of a chronic lower respiratory disease. This procedure allows the doctor to get a better view of the airways and can help diagnose conditions such as asthma and COPD.

Other tests used to diagnose CLRD include the following:

• Pulse oximetry: This test measures the amount of oxygen in the blood. It is often used to diagnose COPD.

• Bronchial provocation tests: These tests measure how the airways react to a certain stimulant, such as cold air or methacholine. They are often used to diagnose asthma.

• Imaging tests: These tests use X-rays or MRIs to look at the lungs. They can help diagnose and monitor lung diseases.

• Lung function tests: These tests measure how well the lungs are working.

• Arterial blood gases: This test measures the amount of oxygen and carbon dioxide in the blood. It can help diagnose and monitor lung diseases.

• Sputum tests: These tests look at a sample of mucus from the lungs to check for bacteria or other signs of infection.

• Lung biopsy: This test involves removing a small sample of tissue from the lungs and examining it under a microscope.

Overall, a combination of diagnostic tests is the best way to diagnose chronic lower respiratory diseases. These tests can help to detect any abnormalities or blockages in the airways, as well as any signs of infection or inflammation, which can be indicative of a chronic lower respiratory disease.

These tests can help diagnose CLRD, but they cannot replace the need for a detailed medical history and physical exam. It is important to see a doctor if you are experiencing any symptoms of CLRD, such as shortness of breath, chest tightness, or wheezing.

The diagnosis of chronic lower respiratory diseases is not always straightforward. It may require multiple tests and careful analysis of the results by a doctor to make an accurate diagnosis. Additionally, some tests may need to be repeated over time to monitor any changes in the condition.

It is important to remember that a chronic lower respiratory disease diagnosis does not necessarily mean that the individual has an incurable condition. With the right combination of medications, lifestyle changes, and other treatments, it is possible to manage the symptoms and improve the individual's quality of life.

If you suspect that you may have a chronic lower respiratory disease, it is important to talk to your doctor about the diagnostic tests that may be necessary. Early diagnosis and treatment help the doctor determine the severity of the disease, the presence of any complications, and the best course of treatment. Patients need to follow their doctor's instructions and get regular

check-ups to ensure that their condition is
being managed properly.

Medical Tests

Medical treatment for chronic lower
respiratory diseases such as COPD, asthma,
and bronchitis focuses on relieving
symptoms, preventing further damage to
the lungs, and preventing exacerbations.
Treatments typically involve a combination
of medications, lifestyle changes, and
breathing exercises.

Medications: Medications are used to
reduce symptoms and improve quality of
life. Long-term medications are used to
control symptoms and reduce inflammation
in the lungs. Common medications used to
treat CLRD include bronchodilators, inhaled
corticosteroids, anticholinergics, and
antibiotics. Bronchodilators help to open up
the airways, allowing more air to flow
through. Inhaled corticosteroids reduce

inflammation in the airways and reduce airway constriction. Anticholinergics help to reduce airway spasms and mucus production. Other medications may be prescribed depending on the type and severity of disease, including antibiotics, inhalers, mucolytic agents, and oxygen therapy.

Lifestyle Changes: Lifestyle changes are important for everyone with CLRD. This includes quitting smoking, avoiding secondhand smoke, exercising regularly, eating a healthy diet, and getting plenty of rest. People with CLRD should also avoid air pollutants, such as smoke or chemicals, and keep their homes free of dust, mold, and pet dander. Making lifestyle changes can help improve symptoms and prevent exacerbations.

Breathing Exercises: Doing breathing exercises can help to improve lung strength and reduce symptoms. These exercises can involve pursed lip breathing, diaphragmatic breathing, and chest breathing.

Other Therapies: In some cases, other therapies may be recommended. Oxygen therapy can help to increase the amount of oxygen in the blood, which can improve breathing and reduce symptoms. Pulmonary rehabilitation can help to improve lung function and exercise tolerance.

In severe cases, surgery or other treatments may be an option. Surgery may be used to remove damaged tissue or to open narrowed airways. However, surgery is not always a viable option and may not provide long-term relief.
Other treatments may include stem cell therapy or lung transplantation.

In addition to medical treatments, there are several other measures that can be taken to manage CLRD. People with CLRD should get regular vaccinations and be mindful of environmental triggers that could worsen their symptoms.

Medical treatment for CLRD is designed to reduce symptoms, improve quality of life, and reduce the risk of complications. Treatment plans can vary depending on the type and severity of the disease and may include medications, lifestyle changes, and other therapies. It is important to work with your doctor to develop a treatment plan that is right for you.

Support from family and friends is also important for those living with a chronic lower respiratory disease. Joining a support group can help provide emotional support and help those living with the condition learn more about the disease and how to manage it. Pulmonary rehabilitation programs are also available to help people with CLRD learn how to better manage their condition.

HOMECARE AND LIFESTYLE MODIFCATION

Living with a chronic lower respiratory disease can be difficult, but with the right treatment and lifestyle changes, it is possible to manage the symptoms and have an improved quality of life.

Home care and lifestyle modification are important components of managing chronic lower respiratory diseases. These strategies can help to reduce the severity and frequency of symptoms, improve quality of life, and delay the progression of the disease. Home care involves self-management of symptoms, with the goal of improving daily functioning. Lifestyle modification involves changes in habits and environment to reduce exposure to triggers like allergens and irritants, as well as to promote activities like exercise, which can improve physical health and psychological well-being. Both home care and lifestyle modification are important in the overall management of chronic lower respiratory diseases.

Nutrition And Exercise

Nutrition is an important part of managing chronic lower respiratory diseases such as chronic obstructive pulmonary disease (COPD), asthma, and bronchitis. Proper nutrition can help to maintain healthy lung function, improve overall well-being, and reduce symptoms. Individuals need to eat that includes plenty of fruits and vegetables, lean proteins, and healthy fats. Foods that are high in antioxidants, omega-3 fatty acids, and vitamin E can help to reduce inflammation and protect the lungs from further damage.

The respiratory system is essential for oxygenation and the exchange of carbon dioxide. People with chronic lower respiratory diseases are at a higher risk for malnutrition because their lungs are not able to process oxygen as efficiently as the lungs of healthy individuals. Poor nutrition can lead to an increased risk of infection, further respiratory complications, and a decreased ability to fight off disease. Therefore, it is essential for them to focus on their nutrition to help improve their overall health and respiratory function.

A well-rounded diet is important to get a variety of nutrients, as different nutrients can help to improve respiratory function and reduce inflammation. A healthy diet should include whole grains, fruits and vegetables, lean proteins, and healthy fats. Eating a variety of foods can help to ensure that a person is getting the essential vitamins and minerals needed for good health. Fruits and vegetables are especially important, as they are rich in antioxidants, which can help to reduce inflammation within the lungs.

You may need to adjust your diet to ensure that your body is getting the nutrients it needs. For example, people with COPD may need to increase their intake of foods that are high in protein and fiber in order to help them maintain a healthy weight. People with asthma may need to watch their intake of foods that can trigger an asthma attack. Additionally, people with bronchitis may need to avoid certain foods that can irritate the airways, such as spicy foods.

In addition to getting a variety of nutrients, it is important for people with chronic lower respiratory diseases to limit their intake of processed foods and sugar. Processed foods are often high in sodium, which can increase fluid retention and further strain the respiratory system. It is also important to limit sugar, as it can lead to weight gain, which can worsen respiratory symptoms.

Eating smaller meals more often can be beneficial for people with chronic lower respiratory diseases. This can help to reduce the symptoms of breathlessness and make it easier to digest the food. Eating slowly and taking time to chew food properly can also help.

Supplements can also be beneficial like Vitamin D, omega-3 fatty acids, and probiotics can all help to support your immune system and reduce inflammation. Speak to your doctor if you're thinking of taking any supplements.

If you're struggling to maintain a healthy weight, you may need to adjust your diet. Speak to your doctor or a dietitian who can help you to create a diet plan that meets your individual needs.

In addition to eating a healthy, balanced diet, people with chronic lower respiratory diseases should also drink plenty of fluids. Staying hydrated helps to thin mucus and makes it easier to breathe. Drinking plenty of water can help to thin mucus, making it easier to expel, and can help the lungs to function more efficiently. It is important to avoid drinking alcohol or caffeinated beverages, as these can dehydrate the body and further strain the respiratory system.

It's important to stay hydrated, so ensure you drink plenty of fluids throughout the day. Water is the best choice, but other fluids such as herbal teas and diluted fruit juices can also be beneficial.

Finally, it is important to note that people with chronic lower respiratory diseases should avoid smoking and secondhand smoke. Smoking can make breathing problems worse and can increase the risk of complications. Additionally, secondhand smoke can also aggravate respiratory symptoms, so it is important to avoid being around people who are smoking.

By following these tips, people with chronic lower respiratory diseases can ensure they are getting the nutrition they need to stay healthy. If you have any questions or concerns, it's important to speak to your doctor.

Exercise

Exercising with chronic lower respiratory diseases (CLRD) can be challenging, but it is an important part of managing your condition. CLRD includes conditions like asthma, COPD, and bronchitis, which can make it difficult to breathe and can cause fatigue. Exercise can help improve your overall health and can even help to reduce symptoms of CLRD.

It is important to start slowly when exercising with CLRD. Begin by walking for

10 minutes a day and gradually increase the amount of time and intensity as you become more comfortable.It is important to listen to your body and take breaks when needed.

It is recommended to talk to your doctor or a physical therapist before starting any new exercise routine. They can help you create a plan that is tailored to your individual needs and abilities. It is important to note that some exercises may be more beneficial than others for people with CLRD.

Low-impact exercises such as walking, biking, and swimming can help improve your cardiovascular health and can help you build endurance. These exercises are good choices for people with CLRD because they are less likely to cause shortness of breath.

Strength training can also be beneficial for people with CLRD. Strength training can help improve muscle strength an endurance, which can help reduce fatigue and make everyday activities easier. It is important to start slowly and use a lighter weight until you become more comfortable.

Yoga and tai chi are great exercises for people with CLRD. These exercises can help improve your breathing and muscle strength, while also helping to reduce stress and tension. These exercises emphasize slow, controlled movements and deep breathing, which can help to reduce shortness of breath.

The key is to start slowly and find activities that you can enjoy and that meet your individual needs. Here are some tips and exercises to help you get started.

1. Warm-up Before Exercise: It's important to warm up before any exercise to help prevent injury. Warm-up activities can include walking, stretching, and light jogging.

2. Aerobic Exercise: Aerobic exercises can help improve lung function and breathing. Examples of aerobic exercises include walking, swimming, and biking.

3. Strength Training: Strength training can help build muscle, which can help improve strength and endurance. Try using light weights or resistance bands for strength training exercises.

4. Balance Training: Balance training exercises can help improve coordination, flexibility, and stability. These exercises can include yoga, tai chi, and simple balance exercises, like standing on one foot.

5. Breathing Exercises: Breathing exercises can help improve lung capacity and breathing efficiency. Examples of breathing exercises include pursed-lip breathing and diaphragmatic breathing.

When exercising with CLRD, it is important to be aware of your breathing. It is important to focus on taking slow, deep breaths and to stop and rest if you are feeling short of breath or tired. It is also important to keep an inhaler or other medications with you at all times in case you experience an exacerbation.

It is important to start slowly and talk to your doctor or physical therapist before starting any new exercise routine. With the right plan and the right attitude, you can find exercises that work for you and help you to maintain your health and quality of life.

Living with a chronic lower respiratory disease can cause a lot of stress and fatigue. Managing these symptoms can be a challenge, but it is possible to find ways to reduce the impact of stress and fatigue on your daily life.

This can lead to a reduction in quality of life and an increase in risk of exacerbations.

Managing Stress And Fatigue

The first step to managing stress and fatigue is to recognize the signs and symptoms. Stress can manifest in many ways such as irritability, difficulty sleeping, difficulty concentrating, and physical tension.
Fatigue can be caused by a variety of factors including lack of sleep, physical activity, or medication side effects. Identifying the symptoms and causes of your stress and fatigue can help you develop strategies to manage it.

Once the causes and triggers of stress and fatigue are identified, there are a number of strategies that can be used to help manage them. These include:

1. Get enough rest. Make sure to get enough rest each day, especially if you're feeling

fatigued. Try to go to bed and wake up at the same time each day and avoid screens close to bedtime. Additionally, taking breaks throughout the day to relax can be beneficial.

2. Create a routine: One way to manage stress and fatigue is to create a routine and stick to it. Setting a daily schedule and trying to stick to it can help you stay organized and manage your energy levels. It can also help you plan for times of rest and relaxation, which can help reduce stress and fatigue. Establishing a regular sleep schedule and trying to stick to it can help ensure that you get enough rest. If you are having trouble sleeping, talk to your doctor about potential solutions.

3. Take some "me" time. Make sure to take some time for yourself each day to relax and unwind. This could include activities such as reading, listening to music, or taking a walk. Limit the amount of time spent on activities

that can be physically taxing, such as housework or gardening.

4. Practice relaxation techniques. Relaxation techniques such as deep breathing, progressive muscle relaxation, and visualization can help to reduce stress and fatigue.

5. Exercise regularly. Exercise can help to reduce stress, improve your mood, and increase your energy levels. However, make sure to talk to your doctor before starting any exercise program.

6. Eat a healthy diet. Eating healthy foods such as fruits, vegetables, and whole grains can help to improve your energy levels and reduce stress. Additionally, drinking plenty of water can help keep your body hydrated and help reduce fatigue.

7. Avoid stimulants. Stimulants such as caffeine and nicotine can increase your stress levels and worsen fatigue.

8. Talk to your doctor. Talk to your doctor about any stress or fatigue that you're experiencing. They may be able to suggest medications or lifestyle changes help you manage your symptoms.

By recognizing the signs and symptoms, creating a routine, finding ways to relax, getting enough sleep and eating a healthy diet, you can reduce the impact of stress and fatigue on your life. Remember to take care of yourself and talk to your doctor if you're feeling overwhelmed.

MANAGEMENT OF CHRONIC LOWER RESPIRATORY

Management of chronic lower respiratory diseases is an important and challenging task for healthcare workers. It requires an individualized approach and ongoing monitoring of the patient's condition to optimize the long-term outcome. This includes effective disease-modifying treatments, lifestyle modifications, and patient education to ensure that the patient has the best possible chance of managing their condition and living a full and active life.

Medications

Fortunately, several drugs on the market can help control the symptoms and spread of these disorders.

A chronic inflammatory condition of the airways known as asthma is characterized by bouts of airway blockage and constriction. The symptoms of this airway narrowing include coughing, wheezing, chest tightness, and shortness of breath. The most often recommended asthma treatments are inhaled corticosteroids. These drugs aid in reducing swelling and inflammation in the airways, which facilitates breathing. To open up the airways and lessen broseveral drugs on the market canre frequently administered. Leukotriene modifiers, methylxanthines, and cromolyn sodium are some more asthma drugs.

The progressive inflammatory lung condition known as a chronic obstructive pulmonary disease (COPD) is characterized by a persistent restriction of airflow in the lungs. Bronchodilators are the primary drugs used to treat COPD because they help to widen the airways and lessen bronchospasm. Long-acting beta-agonists (LABAs) may be given for more severe instances of COPD, although short-acting beta-agonists (SABAs) are typically the first line of COPD treatment. To lessen edema and inflammation in the airways, inhaled anticholinergics and corticosteroids may also be utilized. For severe flare-ups, oral corticosteroids may be administered, and infections may require antibiotics.

Scar tissue builds up in the lungs as a result of the chronic lung disease pulmonary fibrosis, which can make breathing difficult and cause shortness of breath. Immunosuppressants, which lessen pulmonary inflammation, are the principal drugs used to treat pulmonary fibrosis. Prednisone and other corticosteroids, as well as other immunosuppressants like mycophenolate mofetil, azathioprine, and cyclophosphamide, may be included in this group of drugs. Antibiotics may occasionally be prescribed to treat infections.

A long-lasting inflammation of the airways known as chronic bronchitis is characterized by a persistent cough and increased mucus production. The primary drugs used to treat chronic bronchitis are bronchodilators. These drugs lessen bronchospasm and aid in clearing the airways. It is also possible to be prescribed inhaled corticosteroids to treat airway edema and inflammation.

Fortunately, there are several drugs on the market that can help control the symptoms and spread of these disorders.

A chronic inflammatory condition of the airways known as asthma is characterized by bouts of airway blockage and constriction. The symptoms of this airway narrowing include coughing, wheezing, chest tightness, and shortness of breath. The most often recommended asthma treatments are inhaled corticosteroids. These drugs aid in reducing swelling and inflammation in the airways, which facilitates breathing. To open up the airways and lessen bronchospasm, long-acting beta-agonists (LABAs) are frequently administered. Leukotriene modifiers, methylxanthines, and cromolyn sodium are some more asthma drugs.

The progressive inflammatory lung condition known as a chronic obstructive pulmonary disease (COPD) is defined by a persistent restriction of airflow in the lungs. Bronchodilators are the primary drugs used to treat COPD because they help to widen the airways and lessen bronchospasm. Long-acting beta-agonists (LABAs) may be given for more severe instances of COPD, although short-acting beta-agonists (SABAs) are typically the first line of COPD treatment. To lessen edema and inflammation in the airways, inhaled anticholinergics and corticosteroids may also be utilized. For severe flare-ups, oral corticosteroids may be administered, and infections may require antibiotics.

Scar tissue builds up in the lungs as a result of the chronic lung disease pulmonary fibrosis, which can make breathing difficult and cause shortness of breath. Immunosuppressants, which lessen pulmonary inflammation, are the principal drugs used to treat pulmonary fibrosis. Prednisone and other corticosteroids, as well as other immunosuppressants like mycophenolate mofetil, azathioprine, and cyclophosphamide, may be included in this group of drugs. Antibiotics may occasionally be prescribed to treat infections.

A long-lasting inflammation of the airways known as chronic bronchitis is characterized by a persistent cough and increased mucus production. The primary drugs used to treat chronic bronchitis are bronchodilators. These drugs lessen bronchospasm and aid in clearing the airways. It is also possible to be prescribed inhaled corticosteroids to treat airway edema and inflammation.

Other Medications are:

1. Bronchodilators: These medications open up the airways in the lungs, making it easier to breathe. Examples include albuterol, ipratropium, and salmeterol.

2. Corticosteroids: These medications reduce inflammation in the lungs and are often used to treat asthma and COPD. Examples include prednisone, fluticasone, and budesonide.

3. Theophylline: This medication is used to relax the muscles around the airways and is often prescribed for asthma and COPD.

4. Mucolytics: These medications break down mucus in the lungs, making it easier to cough it up. Examples include guaifenesin and dornase alfa.

5. Antibiotics: These medications are used to treat bacterial infections in the lungs. Examples include amoxicillin and azithromycin.

6. Anticholinergics: These medications help reduce spasms in the airways and are often used to treat COPD. Examples include tiotropium and aclidinium.

7. Combination inhalers: These inhalers contain a combination of two or more medications, such as a bronchodilator and a corticosteroid. Examples include Advair, Symbicort, and Breo.

Overall, there are several medications available to help manage the symptoms and progression of chronic lower respiratory diseases. It is important to talk to your doctor about the best treatment plan for your condition

Oxygen Therapy

This becoming increasingly popular for treating chronic lower respiratory diseases, such as COPD, asthma, and cystic fibrosis. Oxygen therapy is the process of breathing in oxygen-enriched air to increase the amount of oxygen in the lungs and bloodstream. This helps to improve breathing and reduce the symptoms of chronic lower respiratory diseases.

Oxygen therapy is usually used in addition to other treatments, such as medications, lifestyle changes, and pulmonary rehabilitation. The goal of oxygen therapy is to increase the amount of oxygen in the bloodstream, which can help reduce symptoms such as shortness of breath, fatigue, and difficulty breathing. Oxygen therapy can also improve exercise tolerance. It can reduce the risk of hospitalization and death, and can improve survival in those with COPD or severe asthma.

Oxygen therapy can be administered in a variety of ways, including continuous or intermittent flow, and pulsed or non-pulsed delivery. The amount of oxygen prescribed and the delivery method used depend on the individual's condition and needs. It is important to note that oxygen therapy should only be prescribed and monitored by a qualified healthcare professional. The most common method is through a nasal cannula, which is a device that delivers oxygen through two small tubes that fit into the nostrils. Oxygen can also be delivered through face masks or by using a machine called a concentrator, which removes nitrogen from the air to increase the amount of oxygen in the air that is breathed in.

Oxygen therapy may also be combined with other treatments, such as bronchodilators, inhaled corticosteroids, and physical therapy, depending on the individual's condition. It is important to note that oxygen therapy should not be used as a substitute for these other treatments, but rather as an adjunct to them.

Oxygen therapy has been proven to help reduce symptoms of chronic lower respiratory diseases. Studies have shown that it can improve exercise capacity and reduce the number of exacerbations or flare-ups of the disease.

Oxygen therapy is generally safe, but there are some risks associated with it. These include dry mouth, nosebleeds, and irritation of the nasal passages. It is also important to note that oxygen therapy can be dangerous if not used properly, as it can lead to hypoxia (low oxygen levels) if too much oxygen is administered.

It is important to talk to your doctor about the risks and benefits of oxygen therapy before starting treatment.

Oxygen therapy is an effective treatment for chronic lower respiratory diseases. It can help reduce symptoms, improve exercise capacity, and reduce the need for hospitalizations. However, it is important to talk to your doctor about the risks and benefits of oxygen therapy before starting treatment.

Pulmonary Rehabilitation

Pulmonary rehabilitation is an effective, evidence-based approach to managing chronic lower respiratory diseases. This comprehensive program of care involves a range of services and interventions designed to improve the quality of life of those living with chronic lower respiratory diseases.

Pulmonary rehabilitation is a holistic approach to care that focuses on the physical, emotional, and psychological needs of the individual.

The program typically consists of a multidisciplinary team of healthcare professionals who work together to develop a personalized plan of care for each individual. This plan may include exercise training, nutritional counseling, education about the disease and its management, psychological support, and other interventions.

The primary goals of pulmonary rehabilitation are to improve the individual's physical and psychological condition, as well as decrease their symptoms and the need for hospitalization.

Through pulmonary rehabilitation, individuals gain improved self-management skills, increased physical activity, improved quality of life, and better symptom management. A variety of techniques are used to accomplish these goals, such as exercise training, breathing techniques, medication management, and education.

Exercise training is a key component of pulmonary rehabilitation. A comprehensive exercise program is designed to improve the individual's physical function and reduce breathlessness. Exercise training also helps with weight control, improves muscle strength, and increases energy levels. Other activities that may be included in the program are breathing control techniques, such as pursed-lip breathing and diaphragmatic breathing. Regular physical activity can improve the strength and endurance of the respiratory muscles, reduce breathlessness and fatigue, and improve overall health and quality of life. Exercise training can also help reduce the risk of exacerbations and hospitalizations.

Nutritional counseling is also an important part of pulmonary rehabilitation. Good nutrition helps to maintain healthy lung function, reduce symptoms, and prevent further complications. Individuals are encouraged to eat a balanced diet with plenty of fruits and vegetables, whole grains, and lean proteins. A balanced diet is essential for CLRD individuals as it can help reduce inflammation and improve overall health. A dietitian can guide the best foods to eat, as well as advise on avoiding certain foods that may bring aggravating symptoms.

Education is a key component of pulmonary rehabilitation. Patients are educated on their condition and the importance of lifestyle changes to reduce symptoms and improve their quality of life. Education also includes information on medications, disease management, and how to live a healthy lifestyle.

Psychological support is an important part of pulmonary rehabilitation. It helps to reduce stress, improve outlook, and provide support for patients and their families. Support systems can also help patients manage their condition and cope with the physical and emotional challenges that come with living with a chronic condition. This can include family members, friends, and healthcare professionals.

Pulmonary rehabilitation is an important part of the treatment plan for individuals with chronic lower respiratory diseases. It is also important to work with a healthcare provider to develop an individualized pulmonary rehabilitation program that meets the patient's lifestyle. If you or someone you know is living with a chronic lower respiratory disease, pulmonary rehabilitation may be an effective way to improve their quality of life.

COPING STRATEGIES FOR CHRONIC LOWER RESPIRATORY DISEASES

Chronic lower respiratory diseases can significantly reduce your quality of life. They can make activities such as walking, talking, and even breathing more difficult. Fortunately, there are many ways to cope with these conditions and improve your overall well-being. Here are some tips for managing chronic lower respiratory diseases.

1. Understand Your Condition: The first step in managing any chronic condition is to understand it. Make sure to familiarize yourself with the symptoms, triggers, and treatments associated with your condition. This knowledge can help you better identify and manage flare-ups and make informed decisions about your treatment plan.

2. Follow Your Treatment Plan: Make sure to consistently follow your doctor's instructions for managing your condition. This includes taking medications as prescribed, attending regular check-ups, and following any lifestyle modifications recommended by your doctor.

Create a plan that includes medication management, exercise and activity, relaxation techniques, and other strategies for managing your symptoms.

3. Exercise: Regular exercise can help improve your physical and mental well-being. Talk to your doctor about what types of physical activity are safe for you to do.

4. Stress Management: Stress can worsen symptoms of CLRD. Developing techniques to manage stress can help reduce symptoms and improve quality of life. Techniques such as deep breathing, meditation, and yoga can be helpful.

5. Get Enough Sleep: Sleep helps the body to heal and repair itself. Getting enough sleep can help reduce stress and improve overall well-being.

6. Good Nutrition: Eating a balanced diet can help keep your body strong and improve your overall health. Eating foods rich in vitamins and minerals can also help rehabilitation.

7. Avoid Triggers: Your doctor can help you identify triggers for your condition, such as smoke, dust, and pollen. Avoiding these triggers can help you manage your disease and reduce flare-ups.

8. Practice Relaxation Techniques: Relaxation techniques, such as deep breathing and meditation, can help reduce stress and anxiety. This can help manage your symptoms and improve your overall well-being.

9. Seek Support: Managing a chronic condition can be difficult, so it's important to reach out for help when needed. Consider joining a support group or talking to a mental health professional. Having a support system of family, friends, and health professionals can help you cope with your condition and improve your quality of life.

10. Participate in pulmonary rehabilitation: Pulmonary rehabilitation programs can provide education, exercise, and support to help you better manage your condition.

11. Seek emotional support. It is normal to experience feelings of fear and anxiety when coping with a chronic condition. Seeking emotional support from a mental health professional can help you cope with the emotional challenges of living with a chronic lower respiratory disease.

12. Complementary Therapies: Complementary therapies such as massage, acupuncture, and aromatherapy can help reduce stress and improve quality of life.

13. Quit Smoking: Smoking is the leading cause of chronic lower respiratory diseases. Quitting smoking can reduce the risk of developing these diseases and can help improve symptoms in those already affected.

Living with a chronic lower respiratory disease can be difficult, but there are strategies that can help. Developing healthy habits and lifestyle changes can help manage symptoms and improve quality of life. Talk to your doctor if you are having difficulty managing your symptoms.

Complementary And Alternative Therapy (CAM)

While there is no cure for CLRD, there is a range of treatments available to help manage symptoms and improve quality of life. Traditional medical treatments such as medications and oxygen therapy may help to manage symptoms, many people are now turning to complementary and alternative therapies to further support their health. Complementary and alternative therapies (CAM) are sometimes used to supplement conventional treatments for CLRD.

Complementary and alternative therapies are non-traditional treatments that are used along with traditional medical care to provide additional support for chronic lower respiratory diseases. These therapies include acupuncture, herbal medicine, massage, and yoga.

• Acupuncture – This traditional Chinese medicine involves inserting very thin needles into specific points on the body to relieve pain and improve respiratory function.   Studies have shown that acupuncture may be beneficial for people living with COPD and other chronic lower respiratory diseases by improving respiratory function and quality of life.

• Herbal medicine – Herbal medicine is the use of plants and plant extracts to treat diseases and can be taken in the form of teas, capsules, and tinctures.   Herbal remedies can be used to reduce inflammation, boost the immune system, and reduce the symptoms of COPD. Herbs such as mullein, elecampane, and marshmallow root are believed to help treat CLRD by reducing inflammation and improving breathing. It is important to speak with a qualified practitioner before taking any herbal remedies in order to ensure safety and effectiveness.

• Yoga – Yoga is a practice that combines physical postures, breathing exercises, and meditation. It can help to improve lung function, reduce stress and anxiety, and improve overall well-being.

• Massage – Massage therapy can help to reduce muscle tension, improve circulation, and reduce stress. Massage can be used to help relax the muscles of the chest and back, which may help improve breathing. Studies have found that massage therapy can improve symptoms of COPD and reduce the need for medication.

• Aromatherapy – Aromatherapy is the practice of using essential oils to improve physical and emotional health. Certain essential oils, such as eucalyptus and peppermint, are believed to help improve breathing and reduce inflammation.

• Hypnosis – Hypnosis is a state of deep relaxation that can help to reduce stress and anxiety. It may also help to reduce the symptoms of CLRD, such as wheezing, coughing, and shortness of breath.

It is crucial to be aware of potential risks and side effects that may be associated with these therapies. With the proper guidance and support, these therapies can help to improve the quality of life and reduce the symptoms of chronic lower respiratory diseases. It is important to remember that CAM therapies are not a substitute for conventional treatments for CLRD. It is also important to talk to your doctor before trying any type of CAM therapy. Although CAM therapies can be beneficial, they may not be suitable for everyone.

RESOURCES AND SUPPORT

Resources and support for chronic lower respiratory diseases can come from a variety of sources. Depending on the severity of the disease, some of the most common include

1. Primary care providers. Your primary care provider can help diagnose your condition and provide guidance on lifestyle changes, medications, and other treatments that may be beneficial. They can also provide referrals to specialists if needed.

2. Respiratory therapists. Respiratory therapists are healthcare professionals who specialize in treating and managing respiratory diseases. They can provide breathing exercises, education, and support to help you better manage your condition.

3. Pulmonologists: Pulmonologists are physicians who specialize in the diagnosis and treatment of respiratory diseases. They can provide more advanced treatments,

such as oxygen therapy, pulmonary rehabilitation, and even surgery.

4. Support groups. Support groups are a great way to connect with other people who are living with the same condition. Through these groups, you can learn coping skills, share experiences, and gain emotional support.

5. Online resources. There are many online resources available to individuals living with chronic lower respiratory diseases. These resources can provide information on treatments, support, and advocacy opportunities.

6. Pulmonary rehabilitation programs. Pulmonary rehabilitation programs are designed to help individuals with chronic lower respiratory diseases improve their overall health and quality of life. These programs typically include exercise, education, and psychosocial support.

By utilizing the resources and support available, individuals with chronic lower respiratory diseases can better manage their condition and achieve better outcomes.

Exercising Tips To Follow For People With CLRD

These exercises are designed to help people with chronic lower respiratory diseases improve their breathing and overall lung health. Be sure to speak with your doctor before starting any exercise program.

1. Heel Slides: Begin by lying on your back on a comfortable surface. Keep your legs straight and slowly slide your heels away from your body. The further away your heels are from your body, the greater the stretch you will feel. Hold for 5-10 seconds and then slowly bring your heels back to the starting position. Repeat 10-15 times.

2. Seated Wall Stretch: Begin by sitting with your back against a wall and your feet flat on the floor. Slowly raise your arms above your head and press your shoulder blades against the wall. Hold this position for 5-10 seconds and then slowly lower your arms back to the starting position. Repeat 10-15 times.

3. Arm Circles: Begin by standing with your feet hip-width apart. Raise your arms out to the sides at shoulder height. Make small, slow circles with your arms for 10-15 seconds. Then reverse the direction of the circles for another 10-15 seconds.

4. Deep Breathing: Begin by finding a comfortable seated position and closing your eyes. Take a deep breath through your nose and hold it for 3-5 seconds. Slowly exhale through your mouth and focus on the sensation of your chest and stomach as the air is released. Repeat this exercise 10-15 times.

5. Neck Stretches: Begin by sitting in a comfortable position. Slowly rotate your head to the right, hold for 5-10 seconds, and then slowly rotate your head to the left. Repeat 10-15 times.

A 7-Day Meal Plan For People Living With CLRD

Day 1

Breakfast: Banana pancakes with almond butter and blueberries
Introduction:
These Banana Pancakes with Almond Butter and Blueberries are a nutritious, delicious and easy-to-make breakfast meal that is perfect for those living with chronic lower respiratory diseases. It is a great way to start your day with a healthy dose of protein and

fiber. The combination of the banana, almond butter and blueberries provides a unique flavor combination that will tantalize the taste buds. This recipe has a prep time of approximately 15 minutes.

Ingredients:
- 2 ripe bananas
- ½ cup whole wheat flour
- 1 cup almond milk
- 1 teaspoon baking powder
- 2 tablespoons almond butter
- ½ cup blueberries
- 1 tablespoon honey
- ¼ teaspoon ground cinnamon
- 1 tablespoon vegetable oil

Preparation Method:
1. In a medium-sized bowl, mash the banana until it is smooth.

2. Add the whole wheat flour, almond milk, baking powder, almond butter, blueberries, honey, cinnamon and vegetable oil to the

mashed banana. Mix all the ingredients until a thick batter is formed.

3. Heat a non-stick skillet over medium heat.

4. Drop spoonfuls of the batter onto the hot skillet. Cook for about 2-3 minutes on each side, until golden brown.

5. Serve the pancakes hot with extra almond butter and blueberries, if desired. Enjoy!

Prep Time: 15 minutes

Lunch: Turkey burger on a whole wheat bun with a side of roasted vegetables

Introduction:
This delicious and healthy turkey burger on a whole wheat bun with a side of roasted vegetables is perfect for those living with chronic lower respiratory diseases. It is an easy and nutritious meal that will give you

all the nutrition you need. The prep time is only 30 minutes, making it a great option for a quick and delicious meal.

Ingredients:

For the burger:
• 1 pound of ground turkey
• 1/4 teaspoon of ground black pepper
• 1/4 teaspoon of garlic powder
• 1/4 teaspoon of onion powder
• 1/4 teaspoon of salt
• 2 tablespoons of olive oil
• 4 whole wheat hamburger buns

For the roasted vegetables:
• 2 cups of diced carrots
• 2 cups of diced zucchini
• 2 cups of diced bell peppers
• 2 tablespoons of olive oil
• 1 teaspoon of garlic powder
• 1/2 teaspoon of salt
• 1/4 teaspoon of black pepper

Preparation:

1. Preheat the oven to 400 degrees F.

2. In a large bowl, mix the ground turkey, black pepper, garlic powder, onion powder, and salt. Form the mixture into four patties.

3. Heat the olive oil in a large skillet over medium-high heat. Add the patties and cook for 4-5 minutes on each side until they are cooked through. Set aside.

4. In a large bowl, combine the carrots, zucchini, bell peppers, olive oil, garlic powder, salt, and black pepper. Toss to coat.

5. Line a baking sheet with parchment paper. Spread the vegetables out in an even layer and roast in the preheated oven for 20 minutes.

6. Toast the buns in the skillet over medium-high heat for 1-2 minutes per side.

7. To assemble the burgers, place a patty on each bun and top with roasted vegetables.

Prep Time: 30 minutes

Dinner: Salmon steak with quinoa and steamed broccoli

Introduction:
This salmon steak with quinoa and steamed broccoli is a healthy, balanced meal that is perfect for those living with chronic lower respiratory diseases. It is high in protein, fiber, and essential vitamins and minerals. The quinoa provides a complex carbohydrate that will keep you feeling full for longer, and the steamed broccoli adds an extra layer of flavor and nutrition. This meal is easy to prepare and can be ready in just 25 minutes.

Ingredients:
- 2 salmon steaks

- 1 cup quinoa
- 2 cups water
- 2 cups broccoli florets
- 2 tablespoons olive oil
- Salt and pepper to taste

Preparation:
1. Start by rinsing the quinoa in a sieve, then transfer it to a medium saucepan. Add the water and bring it to a boil over high heat.

2. Once boiling, reduce the heat to low and simmer for 15 minutes.

3. Meanwhile, heat the olive oil in a large skillet over medium-high heat.

4. Season the salmon with salt and pepper, then place it in the skillet. Cook for 5 minutes per side or until it's cooked through and flaky.

5. When the quinoa is done, fluff it with a fork and season with salt and pepper.

6. Steam the broccoli in a separate pot for 5 minutes or until it's tender.

7. Serve the salmon over the quinoa, topped with steamed broccoli.

Prep Time: 25 minutes

Day 2
Breakfast: Overnight oats with chia seeds, almond milk, and raisins
Introduction:
Overnight oats with chia seeds, almond milk, and raisins is a delicious and nutritious meal that is easy to make and perfect for those living with chronic lower respiratory diseases. It is full of fiber, protein, and healthy fats, and will provide sustained energy throughout the day.

Ingredients:
- ½ cup rolled oats
- 2 tablespoons chia seeds

- ½ cup unsweetened almond milk
- 1 tablespoon honey
- 2 tablespoons raisins

Preparation:
1. In a medium bowl, mix together the oats, chia seeds, almond milk, and honey until combined.
2. Stir in the raisins until evenly distributed.
3. Cover the bowl and place it in the refrigerator overnight.

Prep Time: 5 minutes
Total Time: 8 hours (overnight)

Lunch: Kale and white bean soup with whole grain bread
Introduction
This hearty soup is full of nutritious ingredients like kale, white beans, and whole grain bread. It's a great meal for those managing chronic lower respiratory diseases like COPD and asthma, as it's low in

saturated fat and sodium, and high in fiber and protein.

Ingredients

- 2 tablespoons olive oil
- 1 large onion, diced
- 2 cloves garlic, minced
- 2 carrots, diced
- 2 stalks celery, diced
- 1 teaspoon dried thyme
- 1/2 teaspoon dried oregano
- 1/4 teaspoon smoked paprika
- 1/4 teaspoon black pepper
- 4 cups vegetable broth
- 2 cups cooked white beans
- 2 cups diced potatoes
- 4 cups chopped kale
- 2 tablespoons freshly squeezed lemon juice
- 2 tablespoons chopped fresh parsley
- 4 slices whole grain bread, toasted

Preparation

1. Heat the olive oil in a large pot over medium heat. Add the onion, garlic, carrots, and celery and cook until softened, about 5 minutes.

2. Add the thyme, oregano, smoked paprika, and black pepper and cook for 1 minute.

3. Pour in the vegetable broth and bring it to a boil. Add the white beans, potatoes, and kale and reduce the heat to low. Simmer for 15 minutes, or until the potatoes are tender.

4. Stir in the lemon juice and parsley and season to taste with salt and pepper.

5. Serve the soup with toasted slices of whole-grain bread.

Prep Time: 25 minutes

Dinner: Grilled chicken breast with roasted sweet potatoes and a side of steamed spinach

Introduction:

This delicious, healthy, and easy-to-make grilled chicken breast with roasted sweet potatoes and a side of steamed spinach is a great meal option for people living with chronic lower respiratory disease, as the lean protein and vitamins A and C in the dish can help support the immune system. This dish is also low in sodium, which is important for people with chronic lower respiratory diseases.

Ingredients:

- 2 boneless, skinless chicken breasts
- 2 medium sweet potatoes
- 2 cups of spinach
- 2 tablespoons of olive oil
- ½ teaspoon of garlic powder
- Salt and pepper, to taste

Preparation:

1. Preheat the oven to 400°F.

2. Wash the sweet potatoes and cut them into 1-inch cubes. Place them on a baking sheet and drizzle with the olive oil. Sprinkle with the garlic powder, salt, and pepper and toss to combine. Roast for 20 minutes, flipping the potatoes halfway through.

3. Meanwhile, season the chicken breasts with salt and pepper. Heat a large non-stick skillet over medium-high heat and add the chicken. Cook for 5-7 minutes per side until golden brown and cooked through.

4. Bring a large pot of water to a boil and add the spinach. Boil for 2 minutes, then drain and set aside.

5. Serve the chicken, sweet potatoes, and spinach together.

Prep Time: 30 minutes

Day 3

Breakfast: Greek yogurt with honey and walnuts

Introduction

This delicious and nutritious Greek yogurt with honey and walnuts is the perfect treat for people living with CLRDs (Chronic Lower Respiratory Diseases). It is packed with protein, calcium and healthy fats, making it a satisfying and nutritious snack. With its simple ingredients and easy-to-follow instructions, this recipe is sure to be a hit with all CLRDs!

Ingredients
-1 cup Greek yogurt
-1 tablespoon honey
-1/4 cup walnuts, chopped

Preparation Method
1. In a medium-sized bowl, combine the yogurt and honey and stir until well combined.

2. Add the chopped walnuts to the yogurt mixture and stir until evenly distributed.

3. Serve the yogurt with honey and walnuts immediately and enjoy!

Preparation Time: 5 minutes

Lunch: Quinoa and black bean salad with avocado
Introduction:
This quinoa and black bean salad with avocado is a refreshing and nutritious meal. It is packed with protein, fiber, and healthy fats, making it a great choice for people living with chronic lower respiratory disease. With its delicious combination of

flavors, this dish will make a great lunch or dinner.

Ingredients:
- 1 cup of quinoa
- 1 can of black beans, drained and rinsed
- 1 red bell pepper, diced
- ½ cup of red onion, diced
- 1 avocado, diced
- 2 tablespoons of extra-virgin olive oil
- 2 tablespoons of lime juice
- 1 teaspoon of cumin
- ½ teaspoon of cayenne pepper
- Salt and pepper to taste

Preparation:
1. Cook the quinoa according to the instructions on the package.
2. In a large bowl, combine the cooked quinoa, black beans, red bell pepper, red onion, and avocado.
3. In a small bowl, whisk together the extra-virgin olive oil, lime juice, cumin, and cayenne pepper.

4. Add the dressing to the quinoa mixture and mix until everything is evenly coated.
5. Season with salt and pepper to taste.

Prep Time: 15 minutes

Dinner: Baked tilapia with roasted cauliflower and brown rice

Introduction:
Baked tilapia with roasted cauliflower and brown rice is a nutritious and delicious meal that is perfect for people living with Chronic lower resipatory disease (CLRD). This dish is easy to prepare and is packed with protein, fiber, and essential vitamins and minerals. It can be served as a main course or can be used as part of a larger meal.

Ingredients:
-4 tilapia fillets
-1 head of cauliflower, cut into florets
-1 tablespoon of olive oil
-1 teaspoon of garlic powder

-1 teaspoon of paprika
-1 cup of cooked brown rice
-Salt and pepper to taste

Preparation:
1. Preheat oven to 375 degrees F.
2. Place the cauliflower florets on a baking sheet and drizzle with olive oil. Sprinkle with garlic powder and paprika. Roast in the oven for 15 minutes.
3. Place the tilapia fillets on a separate baking sheet and season with salt and pepper. Bake in the oven for 20 minutes.
4. Serve the tilapia with roasted cauliflower and cooked brown rice.

Prep Time: 25 minutes

Day 4

Breakfast: Egg muffin cups with spinach and feta cheese

Introduction:

This easy and delicious egg muffin cups recipe with spinach and feta cheese is perfect for those living with CLRD (Chronic Lower Respiratory Disease). It is packed with protein, vitamins, and minerals that can help boost your immune system, while providing you with the energy you need to get through the day.

Ingredients:
- 6 large eggs
- 1 cup fresh spinach, chopped
- 1/2 cup crumbled feta cheese
- 1/4 teaspoon salt
- 1/4 teaspoon black pepper
- 1/4 cup milk
- 1/4 cup shredded cheddar cheese
- 2 tablespoons chopped fresh parsley (optional)

Preparation:
1. Preheat oven to 350°F. Grease a 12-cup muffin tin with cooking spray.

2. In a medium bowl, whisk together eggs, spinach, feta cheese, salt, and pepper until combined.

3. Divide the egg mixture evenly among the 12 muffin cups.

4. Pour milk into each muffin cup, covering the egg mixture.

5. Sprinkle with cheddar cheese and parsley (optional).

6. Bake for 20-25 minutes, or until the egg muffins are golden brown and cooked through.

7. Let cool for 5 minutes before serving. Enjoy!

Prep Time: 10 minutes
Cook Time: 25 minutes

Lunch: Veggie wrap with hummus and lettuce

Introduction:
This veggie wrap with hummus and lettuce is a delicious and nutritious meal perfect for

those living with chronic lower respiratory disease. The wrap is full of vegetables, protein, and fiber, making it a great option for a balanced meal. The hummus provides a creamy, savory flavor and the lettuce adds a light and fresh crunch. This wrap is ready in just 10 minutes and is sure to be enjoyed by the whole family.

Ingredients:
- 2 whole grain wraps
- 1/4 cup hummus
- 1/2 cup diced tomatoes
- 1/2 cup diced cucumber
- 1/2 cup diced bell peppers
- 1/4 cup diced red onion
- 1/4 cup shredded carrots
- 1/4 cup finely chopped spinach
- 1/4 cup cooked kidney beans
- 1/4 cup shredded lettuce

Preparation:

1. In a bowl, mix together the tomatoes, cucumber, bell peppers, red onion, carrots, spinach, kidney beans, and lettuce.

2. Spread the hummus evenly onto the wraps.

3. Place the veggie mixture on one of the wraps, spreading it evenly across the wrap.

4. Place the other wrap on top and press down lightly.

5. Cut the wrap in half.

6. Serve and enjoy!

Prep Time: 10 minutes

Dinner: Baked salmon with quinoa and steamed vegetables
Introduction

This baked salmon with quinoa and steamed vegetables is a flavorful and healthy dish that is perfect for people living with or at risk of cardiovascular disease. The combination of quinoa and salmon is rich in protein and heart-healthy fats, while the steamed vegetables provide vitamins and minerals. This recipe is easy to make and ready in under an hour.

Ingredients

• 4 salmon fillets
• ½ cup quinoa
• 2 cups of water
• 2 cups of mixed vegetables (such as broccoli, carrots, and peas)
• 2 tablespoons olive oil
• 2 tablespoons of lemon juice
• 2 cloves of garlic, minced
• 1 teaspoon of dried oregano
• Salt and pepper, to taste

Preparation

1. Preheat oven to 375°F.

2. Place salmon on a baking sheet lined with parchment paper.

3. In a medium saucepan over medium-high heat, add quinoa and water. Bring to a boil, reduce heat to low, and simmer for 15 minutes or until water is absorbed.

4. In a large bowl, combine vegetables with olive oil, lemon juice, garlic, oregano, salt and pepper. Toss to combine.

5. Place vegetables on the baking sheet around the salmon.

6. Bake for 15 minutes.

7. Serve salmon and vegetables over quinoa. Enjoy!

Prep Time: 15 minutes

Cook Time: 45 minutes
Total Time: 1 hour

Day 5
Breakfast: Yogurt parfait with berries and granola
Introduction:
This yogurt parfait with berries and granola is an easy and delicious breakfast or snack option. It's a great source of protein and fiber from the yogurt and granola, and nutrition from the berries. It's also a great way to get creative with whatever fruit is in season or whatever you have in the refrigerator.

Ingredients:
- 2 cups plain Greek yogurt
- 1 cup fresh or frozen berries
- 1/2 cup granola

Preparation:
1. In a bowl, stir together the yogurt and berries.

2. Divide the yogurt between two glasses or jars.

3. Top each jar with 1/4 cup of granola.

4. Serve immediately or store in the refrigerator for up to 4 hours.

Preparation Time: 10 minutes

Lunch: Grilled chicken salad with olive oil and lemon dressing

Introduction:

This Grilled Chicken Salad with Olive Oil and Lemon Dressing is a great, healthy meal for those living with chronic lower respiratory disease. The combination of grilled chicken, fresh vegetables, and a light olive oil and lemon dressing make this salad a flavorful, nutritious meal that can be enjoyed any time of the year.

Ingredients:
- 2 chicken breasts
- 2 tablespoons of olive oil
- 2 tablespoons of lemon juice

- 1 teaspoon of minced garlic
- 1/2 teaspoon of salt
- 1/4 teaspoon of freshly ground black pepper
- 2 cups of mixed greens
- 1/2 cup of cherry tomatoes, halved
- 1/4 cup of diced red onion
- 1/4 cup of sliced cucumber
- 1/4 cup of crumbled feta cheese

Preparation:
1. Preheat a grill to medium-high heat.
2. Rub the chicken breasts with 1 tablespoon of olive oil, and season with salt and pepper.
3. Cook the chicken on the preheated grill for 6-8 minutes per side, or until the internal temperature of the chicken reaches 165°F.
4. Remove the chicken from the grill and let it rest for 5 minutes before slicing.
5. In a small bowl, whisk together the remaining olive oil, lemon juice, garlic, salt, and pepper.

6. In a large bowl, combine the mixed greens, cherry tomatoes, red onion, cucumber, and feta cheese.

7. Drizzle the dressing over the salad and toss to combine.

8. Slice the grilled chicken and add it to the salad.

Prep Time: 15 minutes

Dinner: Shrimp stir fry with brown rice and vegetables

Introduction:
Shrimp stir fry with brown rice and vegetables is a delicious and healthy meal that can be enjoyed by people living with celiac disease. It is a savory and flavorful combination of shrimp, brown rice, and vegetables that can be prepared in just 30 minutes.

Ingredients:
- 1 cup of uncooked brown rice

- 1 lb of peeled and deveined shrimp
- 2 tablespoons of olive oil
- 2 cloves of garlic, minced
- 1 small onion, diced
- 1 red bell pepper, chopped
- 1 cup of mushrooms, sliced
- 2 tablespoons of gluten-free soy sauce
- 2 tablespoons of rice vinegar
- 1 teaspoon of sesame oil
- 2 tablespoons of honey
- Salt and pepper to taste

Preparation:
1. Cook the brown rice according to package directions.
2. Heat the olive oil in a large skillet over medium-high heat.
3. Add the garlic, onion, bell pepper, and mushrooms to the skillet and cook for about 5 minutes until the vegetables are softened.
4. Add the shrimp to the skillet and cook for about 3 minutes until the shrimp is cooked through.

5. Add the cooked rice to the skillet and mix it with the shrimp and vegetables.
6. Add the gluten-free soy sauce, rice vinegar, sesame oil, honey, salt, and pepper to the skillet and mix everything together.
7. Cook for another 3-4 minutes until everything is heated through.

Prep Time: 30 minutes

Day 6

Breakfast: Oatmeal with almond milk, banana, and walnuts
Introduction
This oatmeal with almond milk, banana, and walnuts is a delicious and nutritious breakfast that is perfect for people living with CLRD. It offers a balanced combination of carbohydrates, protein, and healthy fats to power you through the day and provide essential nutrients. This recipe is also vegan and gluten-free.

Ingredients
-1 cup of oats
-1 cup of almond milk
-1 banana, sliced
-2 tablespoons of walnuts
-1 teaspoon of cinnamon
-1 tablespoon of honey (optional)

Preparation
1. In a medium saucepan, bring the almond milk to a boil.

2. Add the oats and reduce the heat to medium-low. Stir occasionally.

3. Once the oats have absorbed the almond milk and become thick and creamy, add the sliced banana, walnuts, and cinnamon.

4. Cook for an additional 5 minutes.

5. Serve hot with a drizzle of honey (optional).

Prep Time: 10 minutes

Lunch: Turkey and veggie wrap with hummus

Introduction

This turkey and veggie wrap with hummus is a delicious and nutritious recipe for people living with chronic lower respiratory disease (CLRD). This wrap is low in sodium, phosphorus, and potassium, making it a great option for those on a renal diet. It packs a great protein punch and is full of healthy veggies. This wrap is perfect for a quick and easy lunch or dinner.

Ingredients

- 4-6 ounces of sliced deli turkey
- 1/2 cup of chopped bell peppers
- 1/2 cup of chopped cucumber
- 1/2 cup of chopped spinach
- 1/4 cup of hummus
- 4-6 whole wheat tortillas

Preparation

1. Heat the tortillas in a skillet or microwave according to package instructions.

2. Spread the hummus on each tortilla.

3. Top with the turkey, bell peppers, cucumber, and spinach.

4. Roll up the tortillas and serve.

Prep Time: 10 minutes

Dinner: Baked salmon with roasted potatoes and asparagus
Introduction:
This delicious and healthy meal is ideal for people living with chronic lower respiratory diseases. It's rich in omega-3s and other essential vitamins, minerals, and antioxidants that can help keep your lungs and heart healthy. The salmon is baked with

a lemon-garlic rub and the potatoes and asparagus are roasted to perfection.

Ingredients:
- 4 salmon fillets, 4-6 oz. each
- ¼ cup fresh squeezed lemon juice
- 2 tablespoons olive oil
- 2 cloves garlic, minced
- 2 teaspoons dried oregano
- 2 teaspoons dried basil
- 2 tablespoons freshly chopped parsley
- 2 tablespoons freshly chopped dill
- 2 pounds potatoes, cut into wedges
- 2 pounds asparagus, cut into 1-inch pieces
- Salt and pepper, to taste

Preparation:
1. Preheat oven to 375°F.
2. In a small bowl, mix together the lemon juice, olive oil, garlic, oregano, basil, parsley, and dill.
3. Place the salmon fillets in a baking dish, and spread the lemon-garlic mixture over them.

4. Place the potatoes and asparagus in a separate baking dish, and season with salt and pepper.

5. Bake the salmon for 15-20 minutes, or until cooked through.

6. Bake the potatoes and asparagus for 20-25 minutes, or until golden brown and tender.

Prep Time: 15 minutes   Cook Time: 40 minutes

Day 7
Breakfast: Smoothie bowl with banana, almond milk, and chia seeds
 Introduction:

Smoothie bowls are a healthy and delicious way to get your daily dose of fruits and other nutritious ingredients. This smoothie bowl is especially great for people living with chronic lower respiratory diseases, as it is packed with antioxidants and other nutrients to help keep your respiratory system healthy. This recipe combines banana, almond milk, and chia seeds to create a yummy and nutritious smoothie bowl that's sure to please.

Ingredients:

-1 banana
-1 cup almond milk
-2 tablespoons chia seeds

Preparation Method:

1. Peel and slice the banana into small pieces.

2. Place the banana pieces into a blender.

3. Pour the almond milk into the blender and blend until the banana is fully blended and the mixture is smooth.

4. Add the chia seeds and blend for an additional 15-30 seconds.

5. Pour the mixture into a bowl and top with your favorite fruits, nuts, and/or seeds.

Prep Time: 5 minutes

Lunch: Veggie burger with a side of sweet potato fries
Introduction:
This veggie burger with a side of sweet potato fries is the perfect meal for people living with chronic lower respiratory diseases. With its healthy and delicious ingredients, this meal is full of vitamins, minerals and antioxidants. The sweet potato fries are an excellent source of dietary fibre and are packed with energy and nutrition. This meal can be prepared in less than 40 minutes and is sure to keep you feeling full and energized.

Ingredients:
- 2 medium sweet potatoes
- 2 tablespoons olive oil
- 1 teaspoon garlic powder
- 1 teaspoon paprika
- 1 teaspoon ground cumin
- 1/2 teaspoon salt
- 1/4 teaspoon ground black pepper
- 1/2 cup cooked quinoa
- 1/2 cup cooked black beans
- 1/4 cup minced red onion
- 2 tablespoons diced red bell pepper
- 2 tablespoons minced fresh parsley
- 1 tablespoon ground flaxseed
- 2 tablespoons almond meal
- 1 teaspoon Worcestershire sauce
- 2 teaspoons Dijon mustard

Preparation:
1. Preheat oven to 400°F.
2. Peel and cut the sweet potatoes into thin wedges. Place them on a baking sheet and drizzle with olive oil. Sprinkle with garlic powder, paprika, cumin, salt and pepper.

3. Bake in the preheated oven for 25 minutes, flipping once halfway through.

4. While the fries are baking, combine the quinoa, black beans, red onion, red bell pepper, parsley, flaxseed, almond meal, Worcestershire sauce, and Dijon mustard in a large bowl. Mix until combined.

5. Form the mixture into 4 patties.

6. Heat a non-stick skillet over medium heat and cook the patties for about 4-5 minutes per side, until golden brown and heated through.

7. Serve the patties with the sweet potato fries.

Prep Time: 40 minutes

Dinner: Grilled chicken breast with quinoa and steamed broccoli

Introduction
This simple and delicious recipe for Grilled Chicken Breast with Quinoa and Steamed Broccoli is perfect for people living with

chronic lower respiratory diseases. It is a nutrient-packed meal that is low in sodium and saturated fat, making it an ideal choice for those looking to improve their health. With just four ingredients and minimal prep time, you can have a nutritious meal ready in no time.

Ingredients
- 4 chicken breasts
- 1 tablespoon olive oil
- 1 cup cooked quinoa
- 2 cups steamed broccoli

Preparation
1. Preheat a grill to medium-high heat.
2. Rub the chicken breasts with he olive oil and place on the grill.
3. Grill the chicken for 6-8 minutes per side, or until the chicken is cooked through.
4. Meanwhile, cook the quinoa according the to package instructions.
5. Steam the broccoli until crisp-tender.

6. Serve the chicken with quinoa and steamed broccoli.

Prep Time: 20 minutes

CONCLUSION

In conclusion, chronic lower respiratory diseases are a serious and ongoing threat to the health of individuals and communities. However, with awareness, education, and proper management, the impact of these debilitating diseases can be minimized. Prevention is key, and this book has provided information on how to recognize the warning signs, manage symptoms, and live a healthier lifestyle. Additionally, this book has outlined the importance of working with healthcare providers to identify and address any underlying conditions that may be contributing to the development of chronic lower respiratory diseases.

Ultimately, it is essential to understand the seriousness of chronic lower respiratory diseases and to take necessary steps to reduce the risk of developing them. By following the advice in this book, individuals can take an active role in their health, and be better prepared to manage any respiratory issues they may experience.

With the right knowledge and precautionary measures, individuals and communities can work together to reduce the burden of chronic lower respiratory diseases and ensure a healthier future.

Printed in Great Britain
by Amazon

39935093R10073